Artificial Intelligence in Modern Laboratory Testing: From Water Quality to Vaccine Potency and Yellow Fever Detection

AUTHOR NAME

Vanisha Saini

Chandigarh University

Dr. Vimulapati Hari Prasad
Chandigarh University

© 2024 Vanisha Saini. All rights reserved. This document and its contents, including but not limited to text, images, and any associated material, are protected by copyright law. No part of this document may be reproduced, distributed, or transmitted in any form or by any means, including photocopying, recording, or other electronic or mechanical methods, without the prior written permission of the author. For permissions, please contact Vanisha Saini directly. Unauthorized use or reproduction of any content from this document is strictly prohibited and may result in legal action..Copyright

© 2024 Author Name

All rights reserved.

ISBN:

DEDICATION

This report is dedicated to all the researchers, scientists, and healthcare professionals who work tirelessly to improve public health and safety. Their commitment to advancing science through innovation inspires us to push the boundaries of technology and knowledge. Special dedication goes to the pioneers of artificial intelligence in healthcare, whose groundbreaking work is revolutionizing how we approach diagnostics, testing, and disease prevention.

CONTENTS

	ACKNOWLEDGEMENT	i
1	INTRODUCTION	4
2	ARS POTENCY TEST	8
3	WATER COMPONENT TEST	13
4	ELISA TEST	18
5	BLOOD TEST	23
6	DPT VACCINE TEST	27
7	ASVS POTENCY TEST	36
8	AIR SAMPLER TEST	41
9	CONCLUSION	45

ACKNOWLEDGMENTS

I would like to express my deepest gratitude to my mentors and colleagues who have guided me through this project. Your invaluable insights and support were essential in bringing this report to life.

A special thanks to the laboratory teams who provided their expertise and access to cutting-edge technology. Your dedication to precision and quality has been instrumental in the successful completion of this work.

I also wish to thank my family and friends for their unwavering encouragement, understanding, and patience during the research and writing process.

Finally, I acknowledge the many contributions of artificial intelligence experts and the developers behind AI platforms, whose innovations have made it possible to apply AI in modern laboratory testing, enhancing the accuracy and efficiency of diagnostics across various fields.

1 CHAPTER
INTRODUCTION

The integration of artificial intelligence (AI) into laboratory testing marks a transformative step in modern science and healthcare. AI, with its ability to analyze vast amounts of data with speed and precision, is rapidly becoming a key player in fields where accuracy and efficiency are crucial. This report focuses on the application of AI in various laboratory tests, including water quality testing, ELISA (Enzyme-Linked Immunosorbent Assay), DPT (Diphtheria, Pertussis, and Tetanus) vaccine potency testing, ASVS (Anti-Snake Venom Serum) potency testing, ARS (Anti-Rabies Serum) potency testing, and Yellow Fever testing. Each of these tests plays a vital role in public health, whether by ensuring the safety of our water, validating vaccine effectiveness, or detecting dangerous infectious diseases. The infusion of AI into these processes not only enhances the speed and accuracy of the tests but also offers new opportunities for innovation in laboratory diagnostics.

Water testing, an essential process for safeguarding public health, involves the analysis of water samples to detect contaminants, pathogens, or chemical substances that may pose risks. Traditional water testing methods can be time-consuming and prone to human error. However, AI-driven systems can automate large portions of this process, from sample analysis to data interpretation. Through machine learning algorithms, AI can detect patterns and anomalies that might escape the human eye, ensuring more reliable results and faster responses to potential health threats. In regions where access to clean water is a critical issue, this technology can make a significant impact by improving the reliability and speed of water safety assessments.

ELISA is another testing method that greatly benefits from AI integration. It is widely used for detecting and quantifying substances such as proteins, antibodies, and hormones. ELISA is crucial in diagnosing diseases like HIV, Lyme disease, and some cancers. While the method is already highly effective, AI has the potential to streamline the process further, minimizing human involvement in tedious procedures, reducing the likelihood of errors, and enhancing the accuracy of results. AI-driven image recognition software can analyze the color changes in ELISA plates more precisely than the human eye, which can significantly improve the sensitivity and specificity of the test.

AI In Laboratory

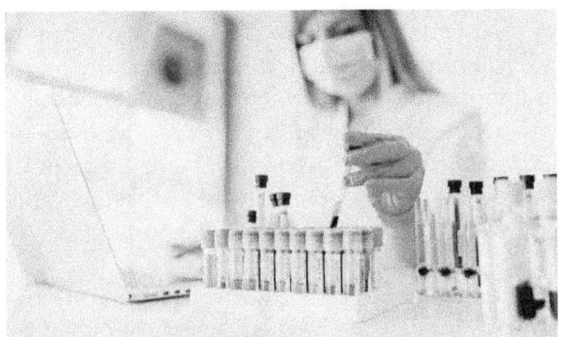

When it comes to vaccine potency testing, such as for the DPT, ASVS, ARS, and Yellow Fever vaccines, AI offers even more remarkable advancements. The potency of vaccines must be meticulously tested to ensure their effectiveness in preventing diseases. Traditionally, these tests can take considerable time and involve complex biological assessments. AI can optimize these processes by analyzing biological responses faster and with greater precision, providing more reliable potency data. This acceleration in testing can be particularly crucial during disease outbreaks, where timely vaccine deployment can save lives.

In addition to efficiency, AI also brings the capability for real-time monitoring and data analysis, allowing for quicker adjustments and improvements to both testing methods and vaccines themselves. In the case of Yellow Fever, an often devastating disease, AI can help in not only testing for the presence of the virus but also in predicting outbreak patterns based on environmental data.

In conclusion, the use of artificial intelligence in laboratory diagnostics represents a paradigm shift in how we approach essential public health challenges. By harnessing the power of AI, we can improve the accuracy, efficiency, and reliability of tests that protect human lives—from the water we drink to the vaccines we rely on. This report explores the practical applications of AI in modern laboratory testing and its potential to revolutionize the future of diagnostics.

As AI continues to advance, its role in laboratory testing will only expand, influencing broader aspects of public health and scientific research. Beyond improving efficiency and accuracy, AI opens the door to predictive diagnostics, where potential health threats can be identified before they fully emerge. By analyzing historical data and identifying trends, AI can help forecast outbreaks of diseases like Yellow Fever or predict fluctuations in water quality, allowing preventive measures to be taken proactively. This capability makes AI not just a tool for improving current testing methods but also a key player in shaping the future of preventive healthcare and epidemiology.

2 CHAPTER
ARS POTENCY TEST

ARS Potency Test: Ensuring the Efficacy of Anti-Rabies Serum

The Anti-Rabies Serum (ARS) Potency Test is a crucial laboratory procedure designed to assess the effectiveness of anti-rabies serum, which is a life-saving treatment for individuals exposed to the rabies virus. Rabies is a highly fatal viral disease that affects the central nervous system and, if left untreated, leads to death in nearly 100% of cases once symptoms appear. Post-exposure prophylaxis (PEP), which includes the administration of rabies vaccine and ARS, is essential to prevent the virus from taking hold. Ensuring the potency of ARS is, therefore, of paramount importance to public health, as its failure could result in ineffective treatment and potential fatalities.

ARS, also known as rabies immunoglobulin (RIG), is derived from the blood plasma of humans or animals that have been immunized against the rabies virus. This serum contains specific antibodies that neutralize the virus, providing passive immunity until the active immunity generated by the rabies vaccine kicks in. The potency of ARS must be tested rigorously to ensure that it contains sufficient levels of these antibodies to neutralize the rabies virus in exposed individuals effectively. 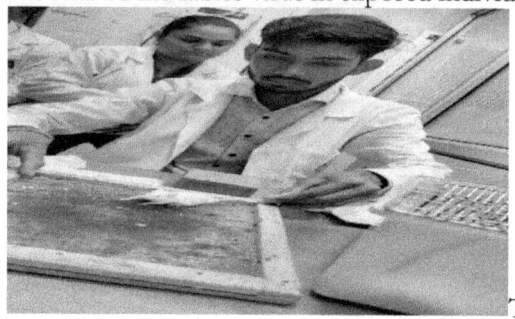 This testing involves evaluating both the concentration and functional capacity of the antibodies present in the serum.

Traditionally, the ARS potency test has been performed using in vivo methods, typically involving animals, such as mice, where the efficacy of the serum is tested by challenging the animals with a lethal dose of rabies virus after treatment with the serum. These tests, while effective, are time-consuming, labor-intensive, and ethically contentious due to the use of live animals. Furthermore, the results of these tests can vary due to biological differences among the test subjects, leading to potential inconsistencies in potency assessments.

Potency	Test Bleed	Manufacturing Bleed	Sublots /final bulk
ARS	>100IU/ml	>150IU/ml	>300IU/ml
ASVS	CV=0.15mg/ml RV=0.15mg/ml KV=0.1mg/ml EV=0.1mg/ml	CV=0.20mg/ml RV=0.20mg/ml KV=0.15mg/ml EV=0.15mg/ml	CV=0.6mg/ml RV=0.6mg/ml KV=0.45mg/ml EV=0.45mg/ml
DATS	>100LF/mg	ActualvalueLF/ml	1000 IU/ml

With the advent of artificial intelligence (AI), there is a growing interest in developing alternative methods for ARS potency testing that are faster, more reliable, and ethically sound. AI has the potential to revolutionize ARS potency testing by automating and improving various aspects of the process, including data analysis, predictive modeling, and even in vitro testing techniques that do not rely on animals. Machine learning algorithms, a subset of AI, can analyze vast datasets from previous potency tests to identify patterns and correlations that may not be immediately apparent to human analysts. This can help optimize the testing process, reducing the time and resources required to validate the efficacy of ARS.

One promising AI-driven approach to ARS potency testing is the development of in vitro assays that can accurately measure the neutralizing activity of antibodies without the need for live animals. These assays typically involve exposing the rabies virus to varying concentrations of ARS in a controlled laboratory environment and using AI to monitor and interpret the interactions. AI can rapidly analyze the data generated by these assays, identifying which concentrations of ARS are most effective at neutralizing the virus and predicting the likely potency of the serum. This process can be completed in a fraction of the time required for traditional in vivo tests and with greater consistency and precision.

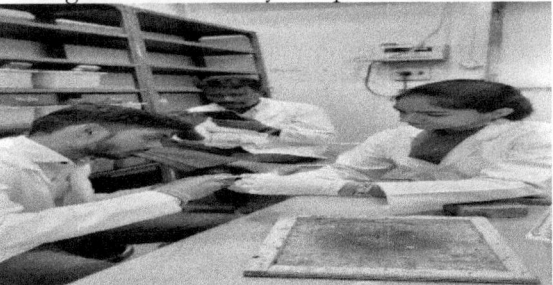

AI can also assist in automating the production and quality control processes for ARS. By analyzing real-time data from production lines, AI can identify potential issues in serum formulation or manufacturing that could affect potency, allowing for immediate corrective actions. This ensures that only high-quality, effective ARS batches reach patients, reducing the risk of treatment failure in critical situations.

Moreover, AI's role in ARS potency testing goes beyond improving current methodologies. It opens the door to predictive analytics that can forecast future rabies outbreaks based on epidemiological data, environmental factors, and human-animal interaction patterns. By anticipating regions where rabies outbreaks are likely to occur, public health officials can ensure that sufficient stocks of potent ARS are available in high-risk areas, thus improving the overall effectiveness of rabies control programs.

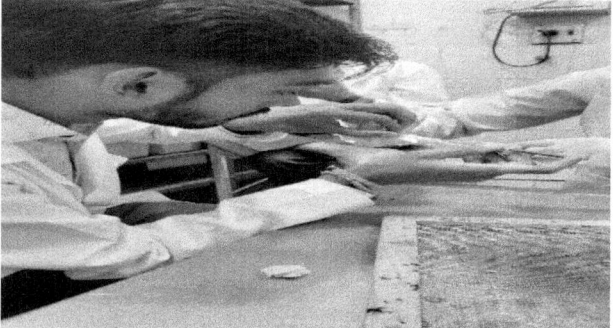

The integration of AI into ARS potency testing is part of a broader trend toward smarter, more efficient laboratory practices. As AI continues to evolve, its application in fields like vaccine potency testing, diagnostic testing, and therapeutic monitoring will only expand. For ARS, the use of AI has the potential to significantly reduce reliance on animal testing, increase the accuracy and speed of potency assessments, and improve public health outcomes by ensuring the availability of potent, life-saving treatments in areas where they are needed most.

3 CHAPTER
WATER COMPONENT TEST

Total Hardness Testing: A Comprehensive Procedure for Water Quality Assessment

Total hardness testing is a critical process in evaluating water quality, focusing primarily on measuring the concentrations of divalent metal ions such as calcium (Ca^{2+}) and magnesium (Mg^{2+}) in water samples. These ions contribute significantly to the "hardness" of water, which has numerous implications for public health, industrial processes, and household water systems. Hard water can cause a variety of issues, from scale formation in pipes and appliances to reduced efficiency in water heaters and boilers. This makes understanding and managing water hardness essential, especially in areas where water quality is a concern.

Importance of Total Hardness Testing

Water hardness refers to the concentration of calcium and magnesium ions dissolved in the water. High hardness levels can lead to mineral buildup in plumbing systems, boilers, and other appliances, reducing their efficiency and lifespan. In addition, hard water can interfere with soap's ability to lather, leading to increased soap consumption in households and industrial cleaning processes. Conversely, soft water, which contains low levels of these minerals, poses fewer challenges in these areas. However, too-soft water can also be problematic, as it may be more corrosive to pipes, leading to metal leaching.

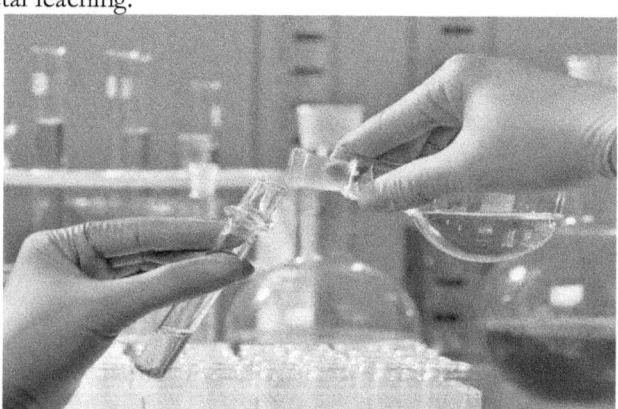

In the context of public health, total hardness testing is crucial. Water that is too hard can pose health risks, such as an increased likelihood of kidney stone formation. At the same time, water with very low mineral content might lack essential nutrients. Therefore, testing for total hardness helps to maintain an optimal balance, ensuring water is both safe for consumption and suitable for industrial and household use.

Step-by-Step Total Hardness Testing Procedure

The total hardness testing procedure involves several steps designed to provide an accurate measurement of calcium and magnesium concentrations in water.

Step 1: Sample Preparation

The process begins with the collection of a 10 mL water

sample. This sample size is standard and sufficient for accurate analysis. The testing begins by adding a spoonful of Reagent 1 to the sample. Reagent 1 typically contains a chelating agent, which is a chemical that binds with calcium and magnesium ions in the water. This chelation process is critical because it prepares the ions for subsequent reactions that will allow their concentrations to be measured.

Step 2: Adding Reagents and Observing Initial Results

Once Reagent 1 has been added, 4-5 drops of a second reagent, Reagent 2, are introduced into the mixture. Reagent 2 serves as a color indicator, which visually signals the presence of hardness ions. After mixing the solution, a color change is observed. In this case, soft water typically remains blue, while hard water turns red. This immediate visual indicator provides a preliminary assessment of the water's hardness level. The red color suggests the presence of significant calcium and magnesium ions, indicating hard water.

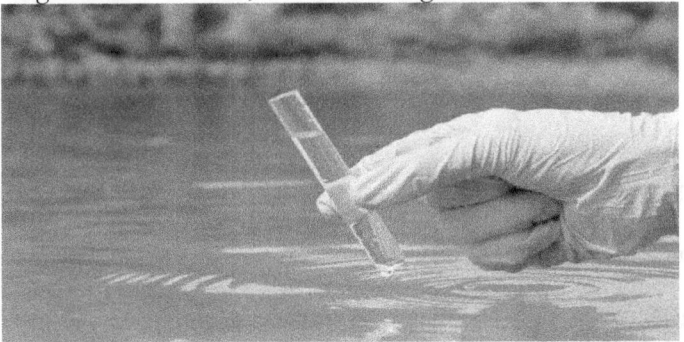

Step 3: Additional Testing Through Titration

If the initial observation reveals hard water (red), further testing is required to quantify the hardness level. To neutralize the hardness ions, Reagent 3 is added drop by drop while the solution is continuously mixed. Each drop of Reagent 3 reacts with the hardness ions, slowly neutralizing their effect. The goal is to continue adding Reagent 3 until the solution changes color from red back to blue. This color change indicates that all hardness ions have been neutralized, signifying that the solution has returned to a soft water state.

Step 4: Calculation of Total Hardness

The number of drops of Reagent 3 required to change the solution back to blue is recorded. This measurement is then used to calculate the total hardness of the water. The total hardness is typically calculated using a simple formula:

$$\text{Total Hardness (mg/L)} = (\text{number of drops of reagent 3}) \times \text{constant factor}$$

The constant factor is usually provided in the testing kit's instructions and varies depending on the specific reagents used. By multiplying the number of drops by this constant, the total hardness of the water, expressed in milligrams per liter (mg/L), can be determined. This quantitative data is crucial for making informed decisions about water treatment.

Significance of Total Hardness Testing

Understanding the hardness level of water is essential for several reasons. For one, it allows households and industries to take appropriate measures to treat water, thus preventing scale buildup in plumbing systems and appliances. Regular hardness testing can extend the life of water heaters, boilers, and dishwashers by reducing the wear and tear caused by mineral deposits.

In industrial settings, the presence of hard water can affect manufacturing processes, particularly in industries where water is used in cooling systems, as a solvent, or in cleaning. Scaling caused by hard water can lead to inefficiencies and increased maintenance costs. Therefore, maintaining optimal hardness levels is not just about appliance longevity but also about operational efficiency.

From a public health perspective, total hardness testing ensures that water meets safety standards for consumption. Water that is too hard may contribute to the formation of kidney stones or other health issues. On the other hand, water that is too soft might lack essential minerals, making it less beneficial for human consumption.

Total hardness testing plays a vital role in water quality management. By following a systematic approach that involves sample preparation, reagent addition, titration, and calculation, water hardness can be accurately assessed. This information is essential for making informed decisions about water treatment and ensuring the health and safety of both industrial processes and public water supplies. As water quality challenges continue to evolve, particularly in the face of environmental changes, maintaining rigorous testing protocols will be key to ensuring sustainable and safe water resources for future generations.

4 CHAPTER
ELISA TEST

The Enzyme-Linked Immunosorbent Assay (ELISA) is a powerful analytical technique used to detect and quantify substances such as proteins, peptides, antibodies, and hormones. This method is widely used in biochemistry, immunology, and diagnostic testing due to its high sensitivity and specificity. ELISA is particularly important in medical diagnostics, research, and pharmaceutical development, allowing for precise measurements of biological molecules in complex mixtures.

Overview of ELISA

ELISA works by using antibodies to specifically detect antigens (target molecules) within a sample. The technique is based on antigen-antibody interactions, where the antibodies bind specifically to their target antigens. The assay is typically conducted in a 96-well plate, where antigens are immobilized on the surface of each well. These plates allow for the simultaneous analysis of multiple samples, which is a key feature of ELISA's efficiency.

The core of the ELISA process involves binding the target antigen to a solid surface, followed by a sequence of reactions involving antibodies that recognize and bind to the antigen. In most ELISA methods, an enzyme is linked to one of the antibodies (or a secondary antibody) that reacts with a substrate to produce a detectable signal, usually a color change. The intensity of this color is directly proportional to the amount of antigen present in the sample. The reaction can be measured using a spectrophotometer, allowing for both qualitative and quantitative analysis.

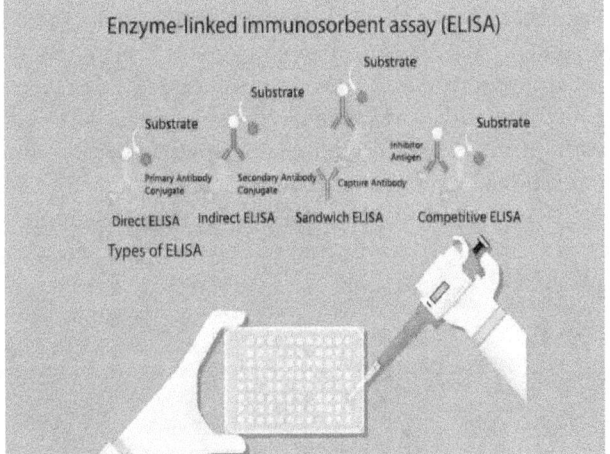

Types of ELISA

There are several types of ELISA, each tailored to specific experimental needs. The most common types include:

Direct ELISA: In a direct ELISA, the antigen is first immobilized on the well plate. Then, an enzyme-conjugated antibody is added, which binds directly to the antigen. This method is simple and quick because it involves fewer steps. However, direct ELISA is less sensitive compared to other ELISA methods because it lacks signal amplification, relying on a single antibody for detection.

Indirect ELISA: Indirect ELISA involves two antibodies. The antigen is coated onto the well plate, and a primary antibody binds to the antigen. After washing, a secondary antibody that is enzyme-linked binds to the primary antibody. This secondary antibody amplifies the signal, making indirect ELISA more sensitive than the direct method. The use of a secondary antibody also makes the assay more versatile, as the same secondary antibody can be used for different primary antibodies.

Sandwich ELISA: Sandwich ELISA is one of the most sensitive and specific forms of the assay. In this method, a capture antibody is first immobilized on the well plate. The sample containing the antigen is added, and the antigen binds to the capture antibody. A detection antibody (also enzyme-linked) is then added to "sandwich" the antigen between the two antibodies. This method is highly specific because it uses two antibodies that recognize different epitopes on the antigen. The sandwich structure enhances detection and makes this method ideal for quantifying low-abundance antigens in complex samples.

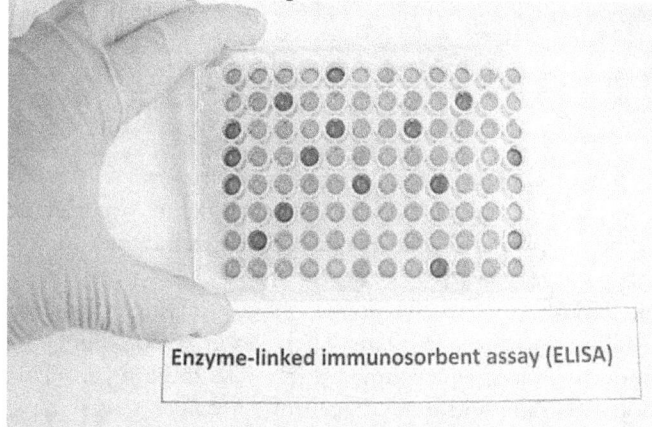

Enzyme-linked immunosorbent assay (ELISA)

Importance of Antigen-Antibody Interaction

The specificity and sensitivity of ELISA are rooted in the antigen-antibody interaction. Antibodies are proteins produced by the immune system that bind specifically to antigens, which are molecules recognized as foreign. In ELISA, this binding is crucial for detecting the presence of the target antigen.

Antigen-antibody interactions are highly specific, ensuring that antibodies bind only to their corresponding antigens, even in samples that contain other proteins or molecules. This allows ELISA to detect even minute quantities of antigens in a sample, making it a sensitive assay for diagnostic and research purposes. The strength of this interaction ensures that ELISA can be applied to a broad range of biological molecules, including proteins, viruses, and hormones.

ELISA Procedure

The procedure of ELISA typically begins with the preparation of the microtiter plate, where the target antigen or capture antibody is immobilized. After this, a blocking agent is added to prevent non-specific binding of proteins. The sample containing the target antigen is introduced, followed by the addition of enzyme-linked antibodies. After washing away unbound substances, a substrate is added to react with the enzyme, producing a detectable color change.

The final step in ELISA involves measuring the intensity of the color produced, which is proportional to the amount of antigen in the sample. This can be done using a spectrophotometer, allowing researchers to quantify the antigen concentration.

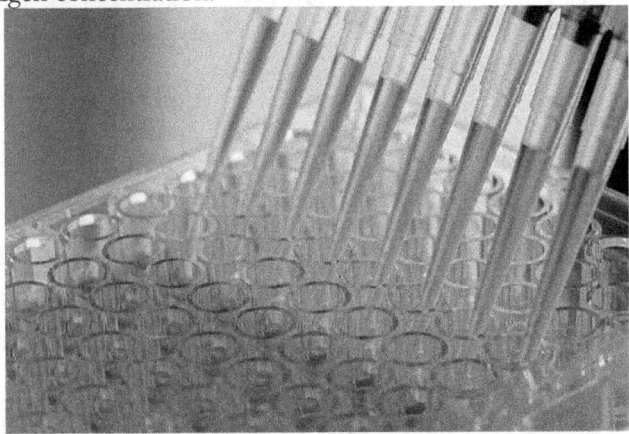

Applications of ELISA

ELISA is a versatile tool used across various fields. In clinical diagnostics, it is commonly used for detecting diseases like HIV, hepatitis, and COVID-19 by identifying specific antibodies or antigens. ELISA is also essential in research laboratories for studying protein expression, immune responses, and other biological processes. Additionally, it is employed in pharmaceutical quality control, where it ensures the consistency and safety of biological products such as vaccines and therapeutic antibodies.

The Enzyme-Linked Immunosorbent Assay (ELISA) is a highly effective technique for detecting and quantifying specific biomolecules. Its foundation on the precise interaction between antigens and antibodies makes it invaluable in diagnostics, research, and pharmaceutical applications. ELISA's versatility—through its different forms, such as direct, indirect, and sandwich assays—allows for tailored approaches to detecting a variety of targets. Its sensitivity, specificity, and ability to handle multiple samples simultaneously have cemented ELISA as a gold standard in biological analysis and diagnostics.

5 CHAPTER
BLOOD TEST

A blood test is a diagnostic tool widely used in healthcare to assess various aspects of a person's health. By analyzing a sample of blood, healthcare providers can gather critical information about an individual's body functions, detect diseases, monitor organ function, and evaluate overall well-being. Blood tests are one of the most common medical tests due to their ability to provide a wealth of information in a relatively simple, non-invasive procedure.

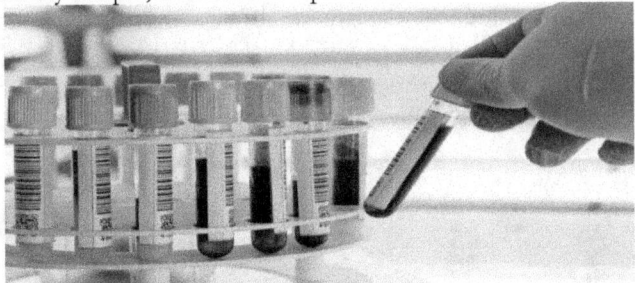

Purpose of Blood Tests

Blood tests serve multiple purposes and are often used as part of routine checkups or to diagnose specific health conditions. They can help detect and monitor diseases, assess the function of vital organs like the liver, kidneys, and heart, evaluate blood sugar and cholesterol levels, and detect infections or immune system problems. Additionally, blood tests are frequently used to monitor the effectiveness of medications or treatments, identify risk factors for certain conditions, and provide insight into nutritional deficiencies or hormone imbalances.

Common Types of Blood Tests

There are several common types of blood tests, each designed to measure specific components of the blood or assess particular health markers.

Complete Blood Count (CBC): A CBC is one of the most routine blood tests performed and provides a comprehensive overview of the cells in the blood. This test measures several components, including.

- ➤ **Red Blood Cells (RBCs)**: RBCs carry oxygen throughout the body. The count, along with measures like hemoglobin and hematocrit, helps diagnose conditions such as anemia or dehydration.

- ➤ **White Blood Cells (WBCs)**: WBCs are part of the immune system and help fight infection. Abnormal levels of WBCs can indicate infections, inflammation, or blood disorders.

- ➤ **Platelets**: These are small cells that help in blood clotting. Low platelet levels may indicate bleeding disorders, while high levels could suggest clotting problems.

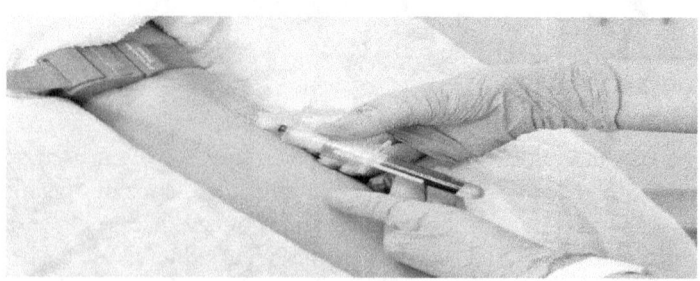

Basic Metabolic Panel (BMP): The BMP assesses the levels of various substances in the blood, such as electrolytes, calcium, and glucose. It also measures kidney function by checking the levels of blood urea nitrogen (BUN) and creatinine. This test helps evaluate conditions like diabetes, kidney disease, and electrolyte imbalances, which are critical for maintaining proper body function.

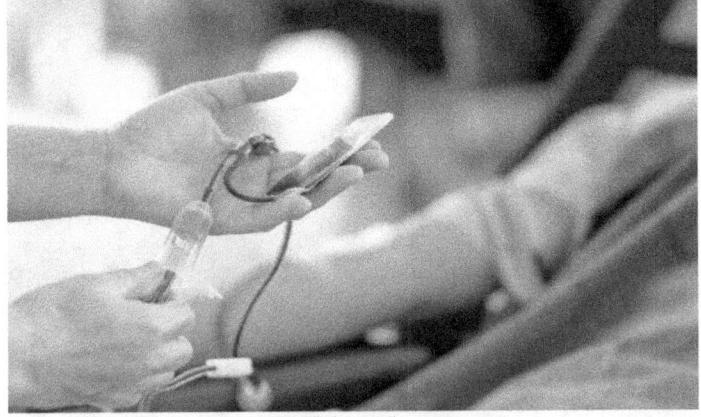

Liver Function Tests (LFTs): These tests measure enzymes and proteins produced by the liver. Elevated levels of liver enzymes such as ALT (alanine transaminase) and AST (aspartate transaminase) can indicate liver damage or inflammation. LFTs are used to diagnose liver conditions like hepatitis, cirrhosis, or liver damage caused by alcohol or medications.

Lipid Panel: A lipid panel measures the levels of cholesterol and triglycerides in the blood. This test provides information about the levels of "good" HDL (high-density lipoprotein) cholesterol, "bad" LDL (low-density lipoprotein) cholesterol, and total cholesterol. High cholesterol levels, particularly LDL, are a major risk factor for cardiovascular diseases such as heart attacks and strokes.

Blood Glucose Test: This test measures the amount of glucose (sugar) in the blood and is crucial for diagnosing and monitoring diabetes. High blood glucose levels (hyperglycemia) can indicate diabetes, while low levels (hypoglycemia) may suggest insulin issues or other metabolic disorders.

Thyroid Function Tests: Blood tests for thyroid function measure hormones such as TSH (thyroid-stimulating hormone), T3 (triiodothyronine), and T4 (thyroxine). These hormones regulate metabolism, and abnormal levels can indicate hypothyroidism (underactive thyroid) or hyperthyroidism (overactive thyroid).

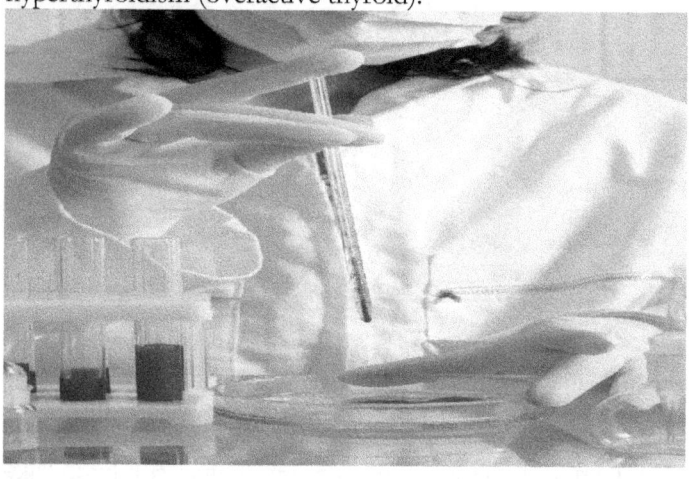

How a Blood Test is Performed
A blood test typically begins with a healthcare professional drawing a small amount of blood from a vein, usually in the arm. The process is called venipuncture. First, a tourniquet is applied to the upper arm to make the veins more prominent, and a needle is inserted into the vein. The blood is collected into a vial or syringe, which is then sent to a laboratory for analysis. In some cases, blood samples may be obtained from a fingertip, especially in point-of-care tests like blood glucose monitoring for diabetics.

The amount of time it takes to get results varies depending on the type of test, ranging from a few minutes for rapid tests to several days for more complex analyses. The results are then interpreted by a healthcare provider who can use them to diagnose conditions, guide treatment decisions, or suggest further testing if needed.

What Blood Tests Reveal

Blood tests can provide insights into several critical health factors, including:

Infection and Inflammation: High white blood cell counts can suggest infection or inflammation, while specific markers like C-reactive protein (CRP) indicate the presence of inflammation in the body.

Organ Function: Blood tests for liver enzymes, kidney markers (BUN and creatinine), and electrolyte levels help assess how well organs are functioning and whether they are being impacted by diseases or medications.

Nutritional Status: Levels of vitamins (such as vitamin D) and minerals (like iron and calcium) in the blood can indicate whether a person is getting adequate nutrition. For example, low iron levels can suggest anemia, while low vitamin D may point to bone health issues.

Blood tests are invaluable diagnostic tools that provide critical insights into a person's health. From detecting infections and diseases to monitoring organ function and medication effectiveness, blood tests are essential for comprehensive healthcare. With the ability to evaluate numerous health markers in a single test, they remain one of the most effective and widely used methods in medical diagnostics.

6 CHAPTER
DPT VACCINE

The DPT vaccine (Diphtheria, Pertussis, Tetanus) is a critical element in childhood immunization programs worldwide, offering protection against three potentially life-threatening bacterial diseases: diphtheria, pertussis (whooping cough), and tetanus. These diseases, caused by different bacteria, can lead to severe complications and even death. The DPT vaccine works by stimulating the immune system through exposure to inactivated toxins (toxoids) and bacterial components, allowing the body to develop immunity without causing the actual disease. By immunizing children early, the vaccine helps prevent these dangerous infections, playing a pivotal role in public health efforts.

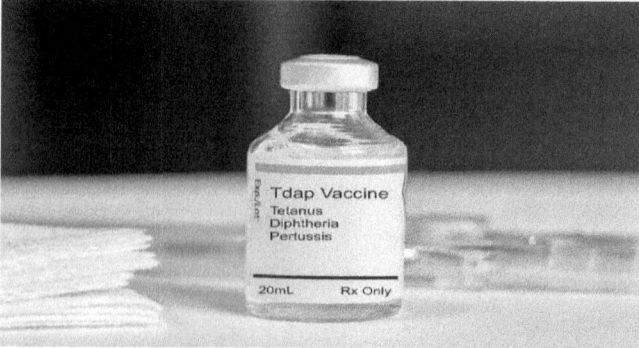

Diphtheria

Diphtheria is caused by the bacterium *Corynebacterium diphtheriae*, which produces an exotoxin responsible for the symptoms of the disease. The hallmark of diphtheria is severe throat inflammation, fever, and the formation of a thick, grayish coating in the throat that can obstruct breathing. The toxin produced by the bacteria can damage tissues, especially in the respiratory tract, and can spread throughout the body, leading to heart and nerve damage. In the DPT vaccine, the diphtheria component is an inactivated form of this toxin. The toxin is treated with formalin, a chemical that neutralizes its harmful effects while preserving its ability to stimulate the immune system. This inactivated toxin, known as a toxoid, primes the body's defenses to recognize and fight the bacteria if exposed in the future, without causing illness.

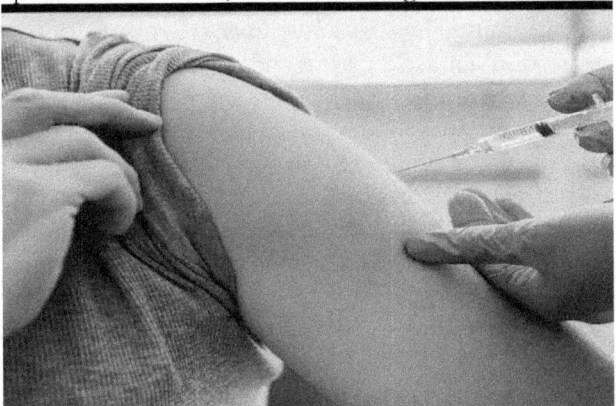

Pertussis (Whooping Cough)

Pertussis, or whooping cough, is caused by *Bordetella pertussis*, a Gram-negative bacterium that releases endotoxins, which are components of its cell wall. Pertussis is a highly contagious respiratory infection that causes severe coughing fits, often followed by a "whooping" sound when inhaling. This disease is particularly dangerous for infants and young children, as it can lead to complications like pneumonia, brain damage, and even death. The pertussis component of the DPT vaccine includes inactivated bacterial fragments, which help the immune system recognize and fight the pathogen. This protection is vital because pertussis can spread quickly through populations, especially in settings where vaccination rates are low.

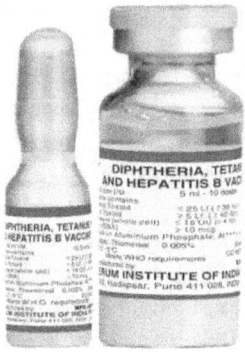

Tetanus

Tetanus, caused by *Clostridium tetani*, is a severe disease that results in painful muscle spasms and stiffness, often leading to "lockjaw," where the muscles of the jaw become rigid and make it difficult to open the mouth. *C. tetani* is a Gram-positive bacterium commonly found in soil, and infection usually occurs through cuts or wounds contaminated with its spores. Once inside the body, the bacterium produces a potent exotoxin called tetanospasmin, which interferes with nerve function and leads to muscle rigidity and spasms. Like diphtheria, the tetanus toxin is chemically inactivated to form a toxoid, which is included in the DPT vaccine. This toxoid trains the immune system to neutralize the toxin, providing protection if a person is exposed to tetanus in the future.

Vaccine Mechanism and Safety

The DPT vaccine works by introducing these inactivated bacterial toxins and fragments into the body, prompting the immune system to produce antibodies against them. This prepares the body to respond quickly and effectively if it encounters the actual bacteria later in life. The vaccine is typically administered in a series of shots during infancy and early childhood, with booster doses later in life to maintain immunity.

To ensure safety and effectiveness, the production of the

DPT vaccine involves several stages of testing and quality control. Tests such as the flocculation test and detoxification test verify that the toxoids used in the vaccine are properly inactivated and cannot cause disease. Specific toxicity tests ensure that the vaccine does not contain harmful levels of toxins. Potency tests are also conducted to confirm that the vaccine triggers a sufficient immune response to protect against diphtheria, pertussis, and tetanus.

Immunization and Public Health

The DPT vaccine is not only important for individual protection but also plays a crucial role in achieving herd immunity. Herd immunity occurs when a large percentage of a population becomes immune to a disease, either through vaccination or prior illness, reducing the likelihood of disease spread. This protects those who cannot receive vaccinations, such as newborns, the elderly, or people with weakened immune systems. In areas with high vaccination rates, the incidence of diphtheria, pertussis, and tetanus has drastically decreased, underscoring the vaccine's effectiveness.

Maintaining high immunization coverage is essential to preventing outbreaks of these diseases. In regions with low vaccination rates, outbreaks of pertussis and other vaccine-preventable diseases still occur, highlighting the ongoing need for widespread vaccination efforts. The DPT vaccine remains a cornerstone of public health initiatives, ensuring that children and communities are protected from these potentially fatal infections.

In conclusion, the DPT vaccine is a highly effective and safe way to prevent diphtheria, pertussis, and tetanus, three severe bacterial infections. By using inactivated toxins and bacterial fragments, the vaccine primes the immune system to recognize and fight these pathogens, significantly reducing the incidence of these diseases. Its role in promoting herd immunity further contributes to public health, particularly in protecting vulnerable populations. The success of the DPT vaccine in controlling these infections underscores its importance in global immunization programs.

7 CHAPTER
ASVS POTENCY TEST

The Anti-Snake Venom Serum (ASVS) potency test is a vital biological assay used to determine the efficacy of antivenom in neutralizing venom from snake bites. Given the potential lethality of venomous snake bites, this test ensures that each batch of ASVS can effectively treat envenomation, helping to prevent death and severe complications. The potency test is conducted by administering venom to lab animals, typically mice, followed by treatment with varying concentrations of ASVS. Observing the survival rates and physiological responses, such as paralysis or hemorrhaging, helps establish the lowest concentration of ASVS required to neutralize the venom. This critical procedure ensures that antivenoms meet stringent safety and efficacy standards before they are distributed for clinical use, playing an essential role in snakebite management and improving public health outcomes.

Materials for the ASVS Potency Test

Several materials are essential to the production and testing of antivenom, including various types of venom, antivenom, and laboratory supplies. Venom samples, such as those from cobra, Russell's viper, krait, and Baro-scaled vipers, are collected and used to stimulate the production of antibodies in animals, usually horses. Controlled doses of venom are injected into these animals, prompting their immune systems to produce antibodies that neutralize the venom's toxins. These antibodies are later extracted, purified, and processed into antivenom.

The production of antivenom requires meticulous attention to detail, including proper storage in sterile, airtight glass vials to avoid contamination. Xylene is used in the laboratory to prepare venom samples for microscopic or biochemical analysis, often as a clearing agent to remove fats or substances that could obstruct the visibility of toxins. Syringes, typically 3ml with 24-gauge needles, are employed for precise injections of venom or ASVS during testing. Saline, an isotonic solution, is another critical component, as it is used to dilute both venom and antivenom solutions, ensuring the proper concentration for safe testing and administration.

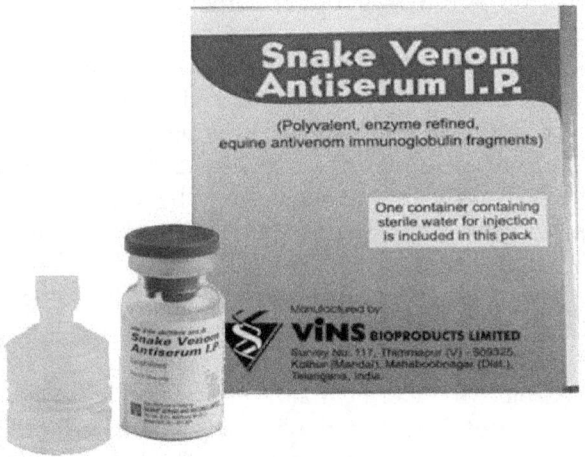

Potency Testing Procedure

The ASVS potency test is structured to assess the interaction between venom and antivenom, focusing on the venom's toxicity and the antivenom's neutralizing ability. The first step is preparing a venom solution, which is made by dissolving powdered snake venom in a solvent, typically saline or distilled water, to create a 10 mg/ml solution. Accurate preparation of this solution ensures consistent venom concentrations, which is crucial for reliable testing outcomes.

A control group is established to observe the effects of venom without antivenom. This control group typically receives 0.125 ml of the venom solution, which may be increased to 0.187 ml to explore the minimal dose-response relationship. This step helps researchers understand how venom behaves at lower doses and establishes a baseline for evaluating the venom's lethal effects. The subsequent experimental doses of venom are incrementally increased, with quantities such as 0.25 ml and 0.312 ml administered to assess the venom's lethal threshold, commonly expressed as the lethal dose 50 (LD50). LD50 refers to the amount of venom required to cause death in 50% of the test animals and is a critical measure for understanding venom toxicity.

Once the venom solution is prepared and tested in control and experimental groups, it is diluted with normal saline to a manageable concentration, ensuring that the venom can be safely tested with antivenom. The diluted venom is then mixed with the ASVS in equal parts—typically 1.5 ml of venom solution and 1.5 ml of antivenom—creating a 3 ml mixture. This step allows for a direct interaction between the venom's toxins and the antibodies in the ASVS, which will ideally neutralize the venom.

Following this, the venom-antivenom mixture is incubated at 22°C (room temperature) for 60 minutes. This incubation period is crucial, as it gives the antibodies in the antivenom time to bind to and neutralize the venom's toxins. The effectiveness of this interaction is evaluated by monitoring the biological responses in the test subjects, such as survival rates or the absence of symptoms like paralysis or bleeding. This step ultimately determines the antivenom's potency and its ability to counteract the venom's effects.

Importance and Implications

The ASVS potency test is indispensable in the production and quality control of antivenom. By assessing the venom's toxicity and determining the minimum effective dose of antivenom, this test ensures that antivenom batches are both safe and effective for treating snakebite victims. The incubation phase, where antibodies bind to venom toxins, is particularly significant because it directly measures the ASVS's neutralizing capacity, which is the foundation of its protective function. Without this test, there would be no guarantee that the ASVS would work effectively in clinical settings, potentially putting lives at risk.

The information gained from these tests is also crucial for improving treatment protocols for snakebites, particularly in regions where venomous snake encounters are common. By refining the methodologies used in ASVS production and potency testing, researchers can enhance the safety and efficacy of antivenoms, contributing to better public health outcomes.

The Anti-Snake Venom Serum (ASVS) potency test is a vital biological assay used to determine the efficacy of antivenom in neutralizing venom from snake bites. Given the potential lethality of venomous snake bites, this test ensures that each batch of ASVS can effectively treat envenomation, helping to prevent death and severe complications. The potency test is conducted by administering venom to lab animals, typically mice, followed by treatment with varying concentrations of ASVS. Observing the survival rates and physiological responses, such as paralysis or hemorrhaging, helps establish the lowest concentration of ASVS required to neutralize the venom. This critical procedure ensures that antivenoms meet stringent safety and efficacy standards before they are distributed for clinical use, playing an essential role in snakebite management and improving public health outcomes.

Materials for the ASVS Potency Test

Several materials are essential to the production and testing of antivenom, including various types of venom, antivenom, and laboratory supplies. Venom samples, such as those from cobra, Russell's viper, krait, and Baro-scaled vipers, are collected and used to stimulate the production of antibodies in animals, usually horses. Controlled doses of venom are injected into these animals, prompting their immune systems to produce antibodies that neutralize the venom's toxins. These antibodies are later extracted, purified, and processed into antivenom.

The production of antivenom requires meticulous attention to detail, including proper storage in sterile, airtight glass vials to avoid contamination. Xylene is used in the laboratory to prepare venom samples for microscopic or biochemical analysis, often as a clearing agent to remove fats or substances that could obstruct the visibility of toxins. Syringes, typically 3ml with 24-gauge needles, are employed for precise injections of venom or ASVS during testing. Saline, an isotonic solution, is another critical component, as it is used to dilute both venom and antivenom solutions, ensuring the proper concentration for safe testing and administration.

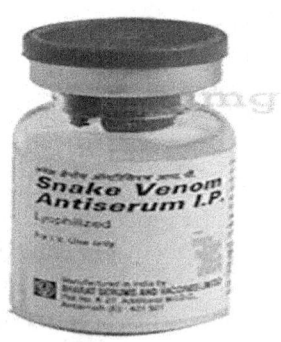

Potency Testing Procedure

The ASVS potency test is structured to assess the interaction between venom and antivenom, focusing on the venom's toxicity and the antivenom's neutralizing ability. The first step is preparing a venom solution, which is made by dissolving powdered snake venom in a solvent, typically saline or distilled water, to create a 10 mg/ml solution. Accurate preparation of this solution ensures consistent venom concentrations, which is crucial for reliable testing outcomes.

A control group is established to observe the effects of venom without antivenom. This control group typically receives 0.125 ml of the venom solution, which may be increased to 0.187 ml to explore the minimal dose-response relationship. This step helps researchers understand how venom behaves at lower doses and establishes a baseline for evaluating the venom's lethal effects. The subsequent experimental doses of venom are incrementally increased, with quantities such as 0.25 ml and 0.312 ml administered to assess the venom's lethal threshold, commonly expressed as the lethal dose 50 (LD50). LD50 refers to the amount of venom required to cause death in 50% of the test animals and is a critical measure for understanding venom toxicity.

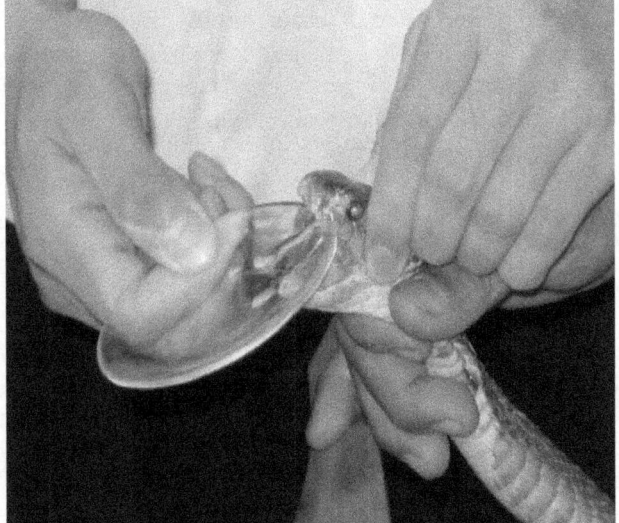

Once the venom solution is prepared and tested in control and experimental groups, it is diluted with normal saline to a manageable concentration, ensuring that the venom can be safely tested with antivenom. The diluted venom is then mixed with the ASVS in equal parts—typically 1.5 ml of venom solution and 1.5 ml of antivenom—creating a 3 ml mixture.

This step allows for a direct interaction between the venom's toxins and the antibodies in the ASVS, which will ideally neutralize the venom.

Following this, the venom-antivenom mixture is incubated at 22°C (room temperature) for 60 minutes. This incubation period is crucial, as it gives the antibodies in the antivenom time to bind to and neutralize the venom's toxins. The effectiveness of this interaction is evaluated by monitoring the biological responses in the test subjects, such as survival rates or the absence of symptoms like paralysis or bleeding. This step ultimately determines the antivenom's potency and its ability to counteract the venom's effects.

Importance and Implications

The ASVS potency test is indispensable in the production and quality control of antivenom. By assessing the venom's toxicity and determining the minimum effective dose of antivenom, this test ensures that antivenom batches are both safe and effective for treating snakebite victims. The incubation phase, where antibodies bind to venom toxins, is particularly significant because it directly measures the ASVS's neutralizing capacity, which is the foundation of its protective function. Without this test, there would be no guarantee that the ASVS would work effectively in clinical settings, potentially putting lives at risk.

The information gained from these tests is also crucial for improving treatment protocols for snakebites, particularly in regions where venomous snake encounters are common. By refining the methodologies used in ASVS production and potency testing, researchers can enhance the safety and efficacy of antivenoms, contributing to better public health outcomes. This is especially important in rural and underserved areas where access to medical care is limited, and snakebites are a frequent cause of morbidity and mortality. Ultimately, the ASVS potency test plays a critical role in saving lives by ensuring that antivenoms are reliable and effective in neutralizing snake venom, thereby reducing the burden of snakebite envenomation.

The Role of Venom in Antivenom Production

Understanding the nature of snake venom is fundamental in developing effective antivenoms. Snake venoms are complex mixtures of proteins and enzymes that vary significantly between species. They can affect multiple physiological systems, including the nervous system, cardiovascular system, and blood coagulation pathways. For instance, neurotoxic venoms can lead to paralysis, while hemotoxic venoms may cause severe hemorrhaging. The ASVS potency test is designed to evaluate how well the antivenom can neutralize these diverse effects, making it imperative that antivenoms are tailored to specific types of venom.

The production of effective antivenoms begins with the careful selection of venom sources. Venom from the most medically significant snakes in a given region is typically chosen for immunization of the animals used to produce antivenom, such as horses or sheep. The antibodies generated in response to the venom exposure are then harvested and purified to create the final antivenom product. This process is critical, as it ensures that the antivenom is not only effective against the venom of a specific snake species but also minimizes potential allergic reactions in patients.

Challenges in Antivenom Development

While the ASVS potency test is a vital part of antivenom production, several challenges remain in the development and distribution of effective antivenoms. One significant challenge is the limited availability of certain antivenoms, particularly in low-resource settings. In many regions, the production of antivenoms can be cost-prohibitive, leading to shortages and inadequate access for patients. Additionally, the variability in snake venom composition means that a one-size-fits-all approach to antivenom development is often insufficient. This variability necessitates ongoing research to ensure that antivenoms are effective against emerging venom types and that they remain potent over time.

Another challenge is the potential for adverse reactions to

antivenom, which can include allergic responses or serum sickness. Such reactions underscore the importance of thorough testing not just for potency but also for safety. The ASVS potency test, along with additional safety assessments, helps to mitigate these risks, ensuring that antivenoms are safe for patient use.

Future Directions

Future advancements in the field of antivenom research and production may include the development of monoclonal antibodies, which are designed to target specific components of venom. This targeted approach could lead to more effective and safer antivenoms, providing better patient outcomes. Additionally, improvements in testing methodologies, including the use of advanced analytical techniques, may enhance the ability to assess both potency and safety in a more comprehensive manner.

Furthermore, educational initiatives aimed at increasing awareness about snakebite prevention and treatment are crucial. Public health campaigns can empower communities with knowledge about the importance of seeking timely medical attention following a snakebite and understanding the role of antivenom in treatment. This, in conjunction with robust testing protocols like the ASVS potency test, can significantly improve the management of snakebite envenomations, ultimately saving lives and enhancing the quality of care for affected individuals.

8 CHAPTER
AIR SAMPLER TEST

The air sampler test is a crucial procedure used to evaluate air quality by measuring the concentration of various airborne particles, microorganisms, gases, and other pollutants. This test is essential in numerous fields, including environmental monitoring, industrial hygiene, occupational safety, and public health. By providing quantitative data on airborne contaminants, air sampler tests help assess potential health risks, enforce compliance with regulatory standards, and inform necessary interventions.

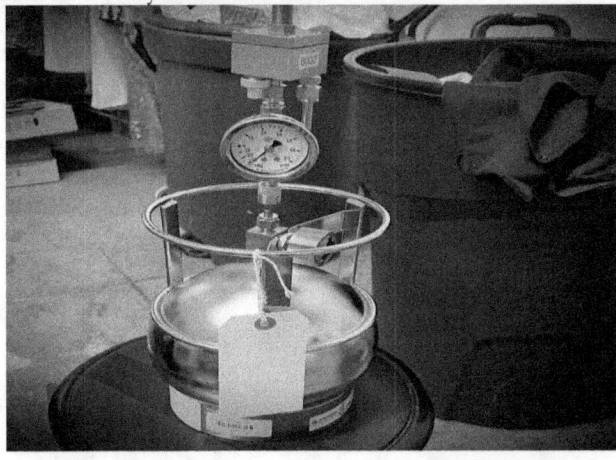

Types of Air Samplers

There are various types of air samplers, each designed for specific applications and pollutants. The most common types include:

Active Samplers: These samplers utilize a pump to draw air through a collection medium (such as filters, sorbent tubes, or impactors) over a specified period. The airflow rate is controlled, allowing for the accurate quantification of airborne substances. Active samplers are often used to measure particulate matter (PM), volatile organic compounds (VOCs), and biological agents.

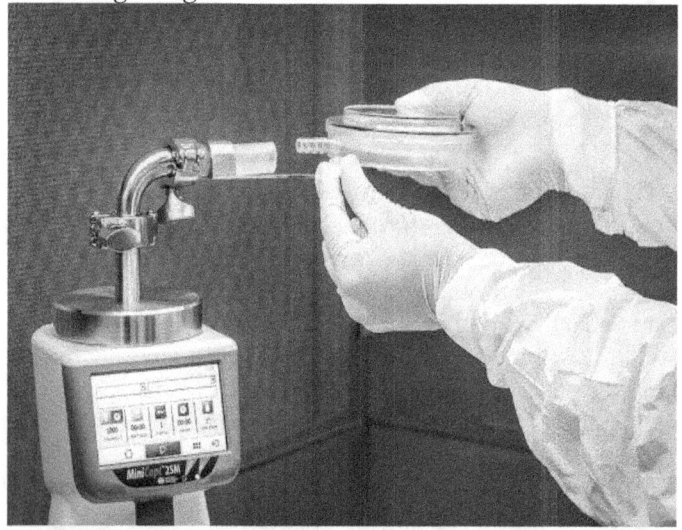

Passive Samplers: Unlike active samplers, passive samplers rely on natural air movement to capture pollutants. These devices typically consist of absorbent materials that trap contaminants over time without the need for a pump. Passive samplers are useful for long-term monitoring of gases or vapors, such as nitrogen dioxide (NO2) or sulfur dioxide (SO2).

Personal Samplers: These portable devices are worn by individuals, providing data on personal exposure to airborne contaminants. Personal samplers can be active or passive and are essential in occupational settings where workers may be exposed to hazardous substances.

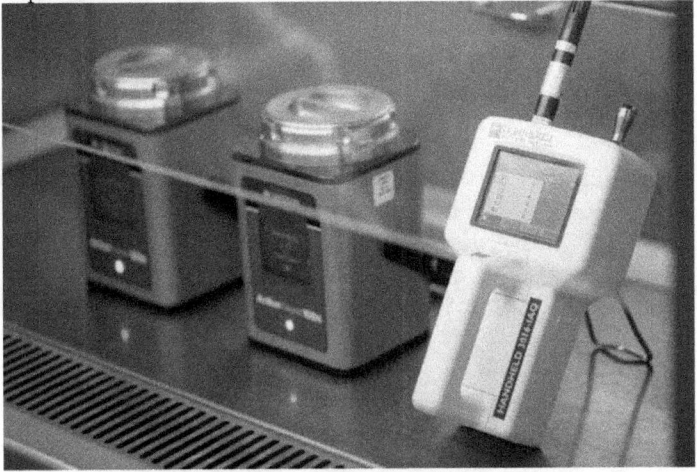

Testing Procedure

The air sampler test involves several critical steps to ensure accurate and reliable results:

Site Selection: Before conducting the test, it is essential to select appropriate locations for sampling. This may include areas near potential sources of pollution, such as industrial facilities, highways, or densely populated zones. Factors such as airflow patterns, surrounding land use, and prevailing weather conditions are considered during site selection.

Equipment Calibration: Accurate measurements require the calibration of air sampling equipment. For active samplers, this includes verifying the flow rate to ensure consistency during sampling. Calibration is typically performed using a flow meter or calibrator, allowing operators to adjust the sampling equipment as needed.

Sampling Duration and Frequency: The duration of sampling is critical and varies based on the specific contaminants being measured and the regulatory guidelines.

Short-term sampling (e.g., 1-24 hours) may be suitable for acute exposure assessments, while long-term sampling (e.g., weeks to months) is often used for chronic exposure evaluations. The frequency of sampling also depends on the intended analysis, with some studies requiring continuous monitoring.

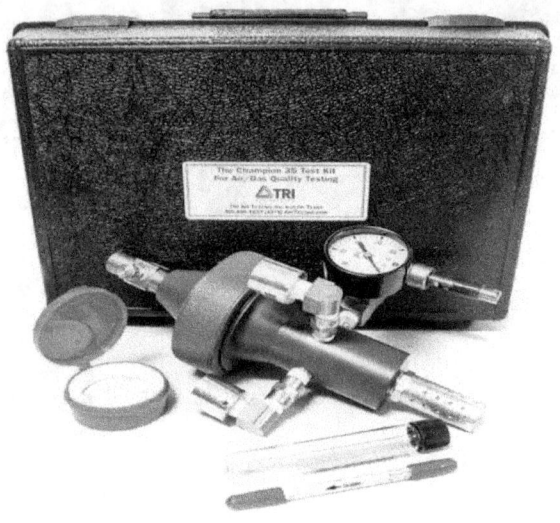

Sample Collection: During the sampling period, the air sampler operates to collect airborne particles or gases on the selected media. For active samplers, the pump continuously draws air through the filter or collection medium. The collected samples are then sealed and transported to a laboratory for analysis.

Analysis and Interpretation: Laboratory analysis of the collected samples typically involves various techniques, such as gravimetric analysis, gas chromatography, or mass spectrometry, depending on the pollutants of interest. The results are quantified and compared against established standards or guidelines to evaluate air quality.

Importance and Applications

The air sampler test is vital for various applications:
- **Environmental Monitoring**: Regular air sampling helps track air quality changes over time, identify pollution sources, and assess the effectiveness of pollution control measures.
- **Occupational Health**: In industrial settings, air samplers evaluate worker exposure to harmful substances, aiding compliance with occupational safety regulations and implementing appropriate safety measures.
- **Public Health**: Air sampling contributes to understanding the health impacts of air pollution on communities, supporting policy decisions, and public health initiatives aimed at improving air quality.

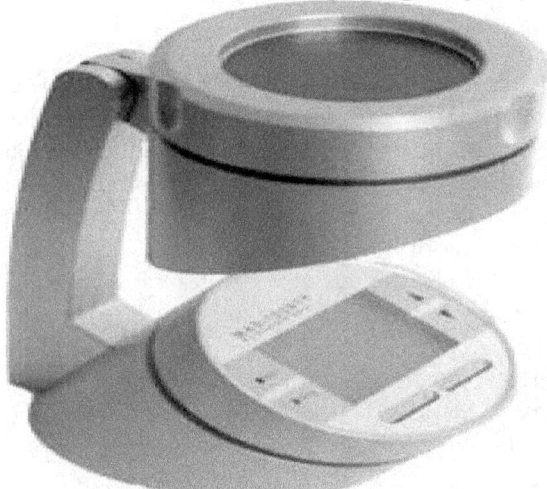

•
  In the air sampler test is an essential tool for assessing and managing air quality, providing critical data to protect public health and the environment. Through systematic sampling, accurate analysis, and robust interpretation, air sampling plays a key role in identifying and mitigating airborne hazards, ultimately fostering healthier living and working conditions.

9 CHAPTER
CONCLUSION

The comprehensive overview of various biological and environmental tests, including the DPT vaccine, ASVS potency test, air sampler test, and their associated methodologies, highlights the pivotal role these assessments play in safeguarding public health and enhancing our understanding of both infectious diseases and environmental impacts. Each of these tests operates within a framework of scientific rigor and quality control, ensuring that the products and measurements derived from them are reliable, safe, and effective. In the context of the DPT vaccine, the intricate processes involved in its formulation, from the careful inactivation of toxins to the rigorous testing for potency and efficacy, exemplify the meticulous nature of vaccine development. The DPT vaccine not only protects individuals from serious diseases like diphtheria, pertussis, and tetanus but also contributes significantly to herd immunity, ultimately reducing the prevalence of these infections in the population. This vaccination strategy is especially crucial in preventing outbreaks and protecting vulnerable groups, such as newborns and those with compromised immune systems. The significance of the DPT vaccine extends beyond individual protection, encompassing a broader public health initiative aimed at minimizing disease burden and promoting overall community well-being. Transitioning to the ASVS potency test, this assay is a critical component in the production of effective anti-snake venoms, addressing a pressing health concern in regions where snake bites pose a significant risk. By evaluating the ability of the antivenom to neutralize specific snake venoms, the potency test ensures that each batch of ASVS meets stringent standards for safety and efficacy.

This test is not only vital for confirming the therapeutic potential of anti-snake venoms but also reinforces the importance of continuous monitoring and quality control in biopharmaceutical production. As snake envenomation can lead to severe morbidity and mortality, the assurance that effective treatments are available can have profound implications for patient outcomes, public health initiatives, and healthcare systems in affected areas. Furthermore, the air sampler test exemplifies the intersection of environmental science and public health. With air quality being an increasingly critical determinant of health outcomes, the ability to accurately monitor airborne pollutants allows for informed decision-making regarding environmental regulations, workplace safety, and public health interventions.

The systematic approach to air sampling, involving precise methodologies and rigorous analytical techniques, enables researchers and policymakers to identify pollution sources, track changes over time, and implement effective strategies to mitigate health risks associated with poor air quality. In urban settings where industrialization and traffic contribute to heightened pollution levels, the role of air sampling becomes especially salient.

By facilitating the collection of data on various pollutants, air sampling not only informs regulatory compliance but also empowers communities to advocate for cleaner air and healthier environments. The integration of citizen science and low-cost air quality sensors further democratizes air monitoring, enabling individuals and organizations to actively engage in efforts to improve air quality and public health outcomes. Collectively, these tests underscore the interconnectedness of vaccination, antivenom production, and environmental monitoring in the broader context of public health. Each test serves a distinct yet complementary purpose, contributing to a holistic approach to health promotion and disease prevention.

The synergy between vaccination programs, effective treatments for venomous snake bites, and robust air quality monitoring initiatives reflects a commitment to safeguarding health across multiple dimensions. As we navigate the complexities of modern public health challenges, the continued investment in research, innovation, and quality control in these testing methodologies remains essential. Advances in technology and scientific understanding will undoubtedly enhance the effectiveness of these tests, paving the way for improved health outcomes and enhanced disease management strategies. Additionally, the emphasis on interdisciplinary collaboration among public health officials, researchers, and communities will be critical in addressing emerging health threats and environmental challenges. By fostering a culture of vigilance and responsiveness, we can better prepare for the evolving landscape of public health, characterized by new pathogens, environmental changes, and shifting health paradigms.

Ultimately, the comprehensive testing of vaccines, antivenoms, and air quality serves as a testament to our collective commitment to health promotion and disease prevention. By prioritizing rigorous testing methodologies, we can ensure that effective interventions are developed and implemented, thus safeguarding the health of individuals and communities alike. This multifaceted approach not only addresses immediate health concerns but also lays the foundation for sustainable health improvements that can transcend generations. As we continue to face the challenges of a rapidly changing world, the integration of innovative testing strategies will be pivotal in ensuring that public health remains at the forefront of our global priorities. In conclusion, the DPT vaccine, ASVS potency test, and air sampler test each represent critical components of a comprehensive public health strategy aimed at preventing diseases, managing health risks, and ensuring a healthier environment for current and future generations.

Through rigorous testing, ongoing research, and collaborative efforts, we can continue to enhance our understanding of health determinants and implement effective interventions that promote well-being across populations. The future of public health will undoubtedly rely on our ability to adapt, innovate, and remain vigilant in our pursuit of health equity and environmental sustainability.

ABOUT THE AUTHOR

Vanisha Saini is a dedicated researcher in the fields of immunology and biochemistry, with a strong focus on vaccine development and therapeutic agent evaluation. With an academic background in biological sciences, she has cultivated a profound interest in understanding the intricate mechanisms underlying immune responses and disease prevention. Her research endeavors encompass a range of critical topics, including the potency testing of anti-snake venom serum, the development and evaluation of vaccines like the DPT vaccine, and the application of diagnostic assays such as ELISA. Vanisha's work aims to bridge the gap between scientific research and public understanding, emphasizing the importance of immunization and therapeutic interventions in enhancing public health outcomes. Through her writing and research, she seeks to disseminate knowledge on emerging biotechnologies and their practical applications in healthcare, fostering greater awareness of the critical role these advancements play in disease prevention and treatment. Passionate about scientific communication, Vanisha is committed to contributing to the advancement of biomedical sciences and improving global health through her findings and insights.

www.ingramcontent.com/pod-product-compliance
Lightning Source LLC
Chambersburg PA
CBHW070419230526
45471CB00006B/2890